MW01504179

QUARANTINED!

HOW TO FEARLESSLY PREPARE FOR, FIGHT, AND SURVIVE A PANDEMIC

PATRICIA L. YODER DC

BARBARA J. SCHNEIDER MS

1

Quarantined!

All Right Reserved.

This book details the authors' personal experiences with and opinions about surviving a pandemic]. The authors are not your healthcare providers.

The statements made about products and services have not been evaluated by the U.S. Food and Drug Administration. They are not intended to diagnose, treat, cure, or prevent any condition or disease. Please consult with your own physician or healthcare specialist regarding the suggestions and recommendations made in this book.

TABLE OF CONTENTS

Introduction

Chapter 1.

Quarantine & Isolation

Chapter 2.

An Ounce of Prevention

Detoxing

Chapter 3.

Bad Habits

Chapter 4.

Finances

Chapter 5.

Supplies

Chapter 6.

First Aid

Chapter 7.

Sanitation

Chapter 8.

Water

Chapter 9.

Travel

Chapter 10.

EMF

Chapter 11.

Communication

Chapter 12.

Stay Calm and Keep This Book Handy

**Other Books By The Authors-
Available on Amazon**

Works Cited

INTRODUCTION

It is all over the news and people are beginning to panic. Viruses have been causing havoc worldwide. People traveling far from home are being detained, individuals and families are facing being quarantined in their homes, hospitals are filling up quickly and there seems to be no end in sight.

There are reports telling us not to worry, and reports telling us to worry. Many newspapers have printed articles "Do not panic or become hysterical". Panic is never good, and neither is living in fear. It is, however, important to be prepared. To be prepared a person acts before an event takes place. That is the reason for this book. It is a simple handbook to help you be ready no matter what type of virus or sickness may come along and disrupt our day to day activities and it does not only applies to pandemics, it applies to any type of manmade or natural disaster that may come our way. Most of us are aware that threats are imminent. The chances of being cut off from supplies, health care and communication are great.

This is not a book that only lists the supplies you need to have on hand in case of catastrophe. It is a book with suggestion on how to live and change your life to survive the world we live in today. It does not matter how much food and water a person has on the shelf, an individual must be physically and mentally prepared to endure unforetold disruptions in life.

We have purposely kept this booklet easy to read and easy to understand. Follow as many of these instructions and ideas as possible and no matter what happens, you will have a solid foundation to stand upon if a pandemic occurs. Remember "DO NOT FEAR!" simply be prepared.

CHAPTER 1.

There is a difference between quarantine and isolation. Below is information obtained from US government pages and the CDC that will inform you about laws. Things can change with an executive order, so use the links provided to keep updated.

Here is an interesting fact from Wikipedia "The word quarantine comes from a seventeenth-century Venetian variant of the Italian quaranta giorni, meaning forty days, the period that all ships were required to be isolated before passengers and crew could go ashore during the Black Death plague epidemic" (Wikipedia, 2020).

The time a person is quarantined varies with the disease, in example, at this time the quarantine for the Corona Virus (COVID-19) is 14 days from the last date of exposure. That is because

14 days is the longest incubation period seen for similar coronaviruses (CDC, FAQS, 2020),.

According to the CDC, releasing a person from isolation in regards to Corona Virus (COVID-19) is made on a case by case basis and includes meeting **all** of the following requirements:

- The patient is free from fever without the use of fever-reducing medications.
- The patient is no longer showing symptoms, including cough.
- The patient has tested negative on at least two consecutive respiratory specimens collected at least 24 hours apart.

QUARANTINE & ISOLATION

Quarantine and isolation are used to protect the public by preventing individuals from being exposed to people who may or not have a contagious disease.

Isolation keeps people with a contagious disease separated from people who are well (Branswell, 2020).

Quarantine separates and restricts the movement of people who were exposed to a contagious disease to verify if they become ill.

The United states has quarantine stations at ports of entry and land border crossing in order to limit infectious diseases from entering and spreading in the United States.

In addition to serving as medical functions, isolation and quarantine also are "police power" functions, derived from the right of the state to take action affecting individuals for the benefit of society. (CDC, 2017)

Federal isolation and quarantine are authorized for these communicable diseases

- Cholera
- Diphtheria
- Infectious tuberculosis
- Plague
- Smallpox
- Yellow fever
- Viral hemorrhagic fevers
- Severe acute respiratory syndromes
- Flu that can cause a pandemic

Federal isolation and quarantine are authorized by Executive Order of the President. The President can revise this list by Executive Order.

STATE, LOCAL, AND TRIBAL LAW

States have police power functions to protect the health, safety, and welfare of persons within their borders. To control the spread of disease within their borders, states have laws to enforce the use of isolation and quarantine.

These laws can vary from state to state and can be specific or broad. In some states, local health authorities implement state law. In most states, breaking a quarantine order is a criminal misdemeanor.

Tribes also have police power authority to take actions that promote the health, safety, and welfare of their own tribal members. Tribal health authorities may enforce their own isolation and quarantine laws within tribal lands, if such laws exist. (CDC, Legal Authorities for Isolation and Quarantine, 2020)

Who Is in Charge?

The federal government:

Acts to prevent the entry of communicable diseases into the United States. Quarantine and isolation may be used at U.S. ports of entry.

Is authorized to take measures to prevent the spread of communicable diseases between states.

- May accept state and local assistance in enforcing federal quarantine.

- May assist state and local authorities in preventing the spread of communicable diseases *(CDC, LEGAL AUTHORITIES FOR ISOLATION AND QUARANTINE, 2020).*

STATE, LOCAL, AND TRIBAL AUTHORITIES

Enforce isolation and quarantine within their borders.

It is possible for federal, state, local, and tribal health authorities to have and use all at the same time separate but coexisting legal quarantine power in certain events. In the event of a conflict, federal law is supreme (CDC, Legal Authorities for Isolation and Quarantine, 2020).

Enforcement

If a quarantinable disease is suspected or identified, CDC may issue a federal isolation or quarantine order.

- Public health authorities at the federal, state, local, and tribal levels may sometimes seek help from police or other law enforcement officers to enforce a public health order.

- U.S. Customs and Border Protection and U.S. Coast Guard officers are authorized to help enforce federal quarantine orders.

- Breaking a federal quarantine order is punishable by fines and imprisonment.

- Federal law allows the conditional release of persons from quarantine if they comply with medical monitoring and surveillance.

In the rare event that a federal order is issued by CDC, those individuals will be provided with an order for quarantine or isolation. You can find an example of a Quarantine Order for Novel Coronavirus   at https://www.cdc.gov/quarantine/pdf/Public-Health-Order Generic FINAL 02-13-2020-p.pdf

The document outlines the rationale of the federal order as well as information on where the individual will be located, quarantine requirements including the length of the order, CDC's legal authority, and information outlining what the individual can expect while under federal order.

You can find all of the laws regarding quarantines at the CDC website https://www.cdc.gov/quarantine/specificlawsregulations.html

(CDC, Legal Authorities for Isolation and Quarantine, 2020)

Will there be a pandemic? There is no way to know for certain. One thing is for certain, stressing over it is not going to help anyone. We can take charge of our lives and choose not to live worried and over what the future may bring. A few proactive steps in the right direction can relieve our concern over the unknown.

CHAPTER 2.

AN OUNCE OF PREVENTION

The biggest defender a person has in their body is the immune system. The main parts of the immune system are white blood cells, antibodies, the complement system, the lymphatic system, the spleen, the thymus, and the bone marrow. The main purpose of your immune system is to protect your body from viruses and bacteria. Your immune system works by recognizing the difference between your body's cells and alien cells, allowing it to destroy any that could be potentially harmful. One of the best ways to fearlessly fight a pandemic is to be healthy by building up your immune system. Here are a few steps to get you started.

- Do not smoke.

- Eat a diet high in fruits and vegetables.
- Exercise regularly.
- Maintain a healthy weight.
- If you drink alcohol, drink only in moderation.
- Get adequate sleep.
- Wash your hands with soap.
- Cook meats thoroughly.
- Minimize stress.
- Avoid sugar.

It is bad enough to be quarantined, you certainly do not want to be sick. There are plenty of ways to avoid getting ill, and we hope the following will be helpful to keep you and your loved ones healthy. Unfortunately, even using the best possible safety measures there is always a chance of infection. A healthy immune system can keep symptoms to a minimum. We suggest seeking out a holistic doctor, chiropractor, functional medicine doctor, or talk to your medical doctor

to help you and your family build up
the immune system.

Exercise

Exercise cannot only prevent chronic
health conditions but can boost
confidence and self-esteem. No matter
what your age, the benefits of exercise
are endless.

Even simple exercises can stimulate
the cardiovascular system, which in
turn, improves all body systems.

Exercise also has emotional and
psychological benefits. For instance,
due to the release of endorphins, a
substance secreted by the brain to
help mask pain and bring a feeling of
complete happiness, exercise can
improve the mood.

Exercise is used as prevention care
and the correct exercises can reduce
pain experienced by those with

arthritis and other diseases that cause the swelling of joints.

Massage

Massage therapy is the use of rubbing, kneading and working muscles and soft tissues in order to bring about healing to the body.

When your body is massaged, circulation improves, and oxygen and other nutrients are brought to the body tissues.

Massage can relieve muscle tension and pain, increase flexibility and mobility, clear lactic acid and other waste and enhance immune function.

The types of massage therapy are Swedish, sports massage, neuromuscular (deep tissue), reflexology and cranial sacral.

TIPS FOR A HEALTHY IMMUNE SYSTEM

ESSENTIAL OILS

- Oregano
- Thyme
- Cinnamon
- Hyssop
- Thieves
- Orange Oil

These oils have been known to boost the immune system and are strong virus fighters. Keep in mind that they are very powerful, and it is best to talk to a practitioner who can recommend the correct ones for you and your family.

HERBAL MEDICINES AND SUPPLEMENTS

Herbal medicine, also called botanical medicine or phytomedicine, refers to the practice of using a plant's seeds, berries, roots, leaves, bark or flowers for medicinal purposes.

Although most herbalists agree that medication is best in emergency situations, they view herbal medicines as **the way for a patient to resist disease**, as well as provide nutritional and **immunological support**. The goal of herbal medication is both prevention and cure.

Some top supplements to a heathy strong immune system:

- **Colloidal Silver** is antibacterial, anti microbial, anti viral and anti inflammatory
- **Zinc**- promotes healthy cell and healing ability
- **B6**- supports blood cells and the nervous system
- **Vitamin C**- powerful antioxidant that fights free radicals

- **Vitamin E**- powerful antioxidant that helps fight infections
- **Elderberry**- boosting immunity. It can protect against infections and bacteria. * It is contraindicated in children with diabetes or anyone with an autoimmune disorder
- **Glutathione** – along with other amazing benefits it supports a strong immune system

HOMEOPATHIC MEDICINE

Homeopathy is an alternative medicine that treats a wide range of health conditions through a practice called the "law of similars." This principle states that a substance that can cause disease in an individual can cure that disease if given in small doses known as homeopathic dilutions.

Homeopathic preparations, called remedies, must be prepared in a certain way, and the dilution used will depend on the symptoms being treated. *(YODER, 2017)*

- **Virex** is a homeopathy from Nutriwest is a great product for fighting viruses
- **Total Bac-T** also from Nutriwest fights bacteria

PRECAUTIONS

- If soap and water are not readily available, use an alcohol-based hand sanitizer with at least 60% alcohol. Always wash hands with soap and water if hands are visibly dirty (CDC, FAQS, 2020) **Keep in mind, hand sanitizers do not kill all germs**.
- Keep hand sanitizer in your car. Use it after pumping gas, going into stores and anytime

you have returned to your car from being in public.
- Wash or sanitize your hands after handling mail.
- Wash all produce well.
- Try not to use public bathrooms.
- Wash your face after being exposed to sick people.
- Change your clothes, especially after work and social gatherings.
- Germs lie on surfaces. Do not lay your purse or bag down on public surfaces, if you do, wipe it down.

WASHING YOUR HANDS

You can help yourself and your loved ones stay healthy by washing your hands often, especially during these key times when you are likely to get and spread germs:

- Before, during, and after preparing food.

- Before eating food.
- Before and after caring for someone at home who is sick with vomiting or diarrhea.
- Before and after treating a cut or wound.
- After using the toilet.
- After changing diapers or cleaning up a child who has used the toilet.
- After blowing your nose, coughing, or sneezing.
- After touching an animal, animal feed, or animal waste.
- After handling pet food or pet treats.
- After touching garbage (CDC, FAQS, 2020).
- Avoid close contact with people who are sick.
- Avoid touching your eyes, nose, and mouth.
- Stay home when you are sick.
- Cover your cough or sneeze with a tissue, then throw the tissue in the trash.

- Clean and disinfect frequently touched objects and surfaces using a regular household cleaning spray or wipe.
- Use a facemask when necessary.
- CDC does not recommend that people who are well wear a facemask to protect themselves from respiratory diseases, including COVID-19. (CDC, FAQS, 2020).
- Facemasks should be used by people who show symptoms of COVID-19 to help prevent the spread of the disease to others. The use of facemasks is also crucial for health workers and people who are taking care of someone in close settings (at home or in a health care facility). (CDC, FAQS, 2020)
- Wash your hands often with soap and water for at least 20 seconds, especially after going to the bathroom; before eating;

and after blowing your nose, coughing, or sneezing (CDC, FAQS, 2020).

Keep in mind that soap and water is usually the best way to get rid of germs. If you do not have access to soap and water use alcohol bases hand sanitizer with at least 60% alcohol.

Hand sanitizer can reduce the number of germs on your hands, but they do not get rid of all types of germs. When hands are visibly dirty that may not be as effective. They also do not remove pesticides, heavy metals and harmful chemicals. (Branswell, 2020)

FACEMASKS

A face mask can protect you from contracting a cold, flu or other virus -- just make sure you get the right kind and use it correctly. Wearing a mask is more for people already showing symptoms of viruses and their caregivers than for people trying to prevent it

The Centers for Disease Control and Prevention said it "does not recommend that people who are well wear a facemask to protect themselves from respiratory diseases, including COVID-19," referring to the disease caused by the new coronavirus. Rather, experts caution that putting on a face mask without proper fitting and training could actually increase your risk.

Disposable face masks block large particles from entering your mouth, while a more tight-fitting N95 respirator mask is far more effective at shielding you from airborne illnesses. Both of these masks *can* help protect you from getting a viral infection.

A face mask's main purpose is to keep out the liquid of an infected person's sneeze or cough from entering your mouth or nose. Wearing one can protect you from getting sick if you're in close contact with someone who is ill and also help prevent you from spreading your illness to someone else. Face masks can also help prevent hand-to-mouth viral transmissions, because you can't directly touch your own mouth while wearing one. However, **virologists say that surgical face masks cannot block airborne viruses from entering your body**. For that you'll need a respirator, a tight-fitting protective device worn around the face. When people say "respirator", they're usually referring to the N95 respirator, which gets its name from the fact that it blocks at least 95% of tiny particles. Several brands manufacture N95 respirators, and they come in all different sizes. When shopping for this kind of mask, be sure the packaging says "N95" --

some masks will only say "respirator," but if they aren't marked as N95, you won't get the full level of protection. Also, the masks can be highly effective in preventing viral illnesses, but only in people who actually wore the masks correctly, which is rare.

N95 masks are difficult to put on for people who aren't medical professionals. If you've put the mask on right, it gets hot and stuffy, so a lot of people take it off before it can do any good. They can also be uncomfortable and exhausting to use over time. They're not designed to be worn eight hours a day."

If you don't have access to an N95 mask, a surgical face mask will be sufficient. Keep in mind you will get less protection from airborne viruses if you wear a surgical mask although cloth surgical masks are not helpful at all.

If you do decide to wear a mask, it's important to note that face masks have a very specific lifespan. While there are some with longer lifespans or that have replaceable filters, the most common face masks on the market are disposable and single use. Each one of those is only good for a few hours. To make sure you are using them effectively, there are videos on the internet that can show you how to properly use them (Banse, 2018) .

DETOXING

To keep a healthy immune system, we must get rid of the toxins in our bodies. Following are some ideas to rid our bodies of toxins.

Infrared Saunas:

Far infrared saunas (FIR) provides many of the health benefits of natural sunlight without any of the dangerous effects of solar radiation. Traditional steam saunas raise the temperature of the air to a very high level within the chamber to warm the body. Some people have difficulty breathing in this extremely warm air. FIR saunas work differently Instead of heating the air within the enclosure, FIR saunas heat the body directly. The result is a lower power bill and deeper tissue penetration. In the FIR sauna, the body perspires and receives all the healthy benefits but avoids the harmful and extremely hot air of a traditional steam sauna. FIR saunas are safe for all ages. Some people do not perspire for the first 4 to 6 sessions, it is as though their body has to be trained to sweat.

Benefits from Infrared Saunas include:

Better circulation and increased energy: The saunas emits FIR energy that is absorbed by human cells, causing a physical phenomenon called "resonance". Thus, the cellular activities are instantly invigorated, resulting in a better blood circulation and an overall improved metabolism.

Weight loss: FIR Sauna heat therapy can aid in weight loss by speeding up the metabolic process of vital organs and endocrine glans resulting in substantial caloric loss in a sauna heat session.

Cardiovascular health: The FIR sauna increases heart rate and blood circulation, crucial to maintaining one's health. The heart rate increases as more blood flow is diverted from the inner organs towards the extremities of the skin, without elevating blood pressure.

Detoxification: The skin is often referred to as the 3rd kidney, because it is believed to be responsible for elimination 30% of the body's waste. It can help eliminate chemicals and heavy metals from the body.

Stress Reduction and Relaxation: FIR Sauna heat treatment before a massage also helps prepare a client by creating an overall relaxing effect. It loosens the muscle tissue so the therapist can do a more thorough and effective massage.

Skin Beautification: FIR Sauna heat therapy allows increased blood circulation to carry great amounts of nutrients to the skin, thus promoting healthy tone and texture. It helps the skin to stay soft and eliminates dry skin.

Improved Immune System: A FIR heat treatment in the early stages of a cold or flu has been known to stop the disease before the symptoms occur.

The Infrared Sauna that we prefer and use is from High Tech Health (800) 794-5355

Coffee Enemas:

Coffee enemas are powerful detoxifiers, due to some amazing compounds within the coffee that stimulate the liver to produce Glutathione S transferase, a chemical which is known to be the master detoxifier in our bodies. Glutathione S transferase binds to toxins and the toxins are then released out of the body along with the coffee.

Note organic coffee should be used not commercial coffee.

Reasons on why you should try a coffee enema:

- Reduces levels of toxicity by up to 600%

- Cleans and heals the colon, improving peristalsis.
- Increases energy levels, improves mental clarity and mood
- Helps with depression, bad moods, sluggishness
- Helps eliminate parasites and candida
- Improves digestion bile flow eases bloating
- Detoxifies the liver and helps repair the liver
- Can help heal chronic health conditions (along with eating a whole food diet)
- Helps ease "die off" or detox reactions during periods of fasting or juice fasting, cleansing or healing
- Used regularly for healing in cancer patients

You can buy an enema kit online. Buy some premium ground ORGANIC coffee beans and keep them in the freezer until you need to use the coffee.

Baths of Detoxification

Epsom salts and Ginger: This bath opens pores and eliminates toxins and also helps to eliminate pain. One cup Epsom salts and 2 tablespoons of ginger stirred in a cup of water first. Then added to bath is beneficial Do not remain in tub for more than 30 minutes

Salt and Baking Soda: This bath counteracts the effects of radiation, whether from x-rays or cancer radiation treatments, fallout from the atmosphere or television radiation. Add one cup of baking soda and one to two cups ordinary coarse salt, Epsom salts or seal salt to a tub of water. You can soak for 20 minutes

Apple Cider Vinegar bath: This is used when the body is too acidic. This is a quick way of restoring the acid-alkaline balance. Use one cup to 2 quarts of 100% organic apple cider vinegar to a bathtub of warm water. Soak 40 to 45 minutes. This is excellent for excess uric acid in the body and is especially helpful for the joints and in conditions such as arthritis, bursitis, tendonitis and gout.

Detoxification using supplements:

Through muscle testing we can detect if an organ needs supplementation and or drainage. It is very important to give supplements to the organ if needed and the proper drainage so the body can heal without toxic side effects. Drainage is very important when clearing out fungus or parasites.

Thymus thump

The Thymus Thump can assist to neutralize negative energy, exude calm, revamp energy, support healing and vibrant health, and **boost your immune system.** It is simple but very effective energy technique involves tapping, thumping or scratching on the thymus point.

The thymus gland cannot be felt from the outside of the body. This is because it is located behind the sternum, also called the breastbone. You can thump in the middle of your chest with your fist (think Tarzan). Or, you may want to rub softly or firmly or scratch with four fingers of your hand. Do this for about 20 seconds and breathe deeply in and out.

Platefuls of vitamin C rich foods like dark leafy greens, Brussels sprouts, kiwi fruit, broccoli, and berries protect the thymus gland, a vital immune system organ.

CLEANSING

We also suggest that a person cleanses out toxins and parasites by doing a gut and liver cleanse once a year. There are many to choose from and your practitioner can guide you.

Also, heavy metals and fungus and be detoxed with the aid of supplements (Yoder, 2017).

OTHER METHODS

There are other alternative methods to aid your immune system. We personally use The True Rife daily. You can research this machine at www.truerife.com The machine is not FDA approved and there are no claims of diagnosis or treatments. The choice is yours alone.

CHAPTER 3.

BAD HABITS

We all have bad habits that can make us sick and challenge our immune system. If you or your family members are often ill, it is time to look at your lifestyle. Some of these habits are very addicting and if a person cannot get out to purchase such things as cigarettes, alcohol or recreational drugs, withdrawals can take over. Why not start today, to alleviate yourself from these habits. This is something to think about before disaster strikes. A step at a time in the right direction will help you build up your immune system and be good for your mental health. We have found that it takes 21 days to break a habit.

Besides those mentioned above there are other bad habits that we need to replace with good habits to stay healthy and to help keep others healthy.

DO NOT GO OUT SICK

It is not always easy to stay home when you are ill. Life goes on. The problem is when you are sick with a cold, flu or other contagious disease, you are spreading it to others.

We all need our paycheck and sad to say often if we stay home, we could lose our jobs. Many businesses require a doctor's note to receive paid sick days. Some people do not have insurance and it is a financial hardship to go to the doctor. No matter what, fess up. Do not go to work with a cold feigning "allergies". Let others know so they can take precautions. Wear a mask. Stay away from co-workers. Do not make stops and run errands on the way to and from work.

If you are sick, skip church, meetings and social gatherings. Do not cook food and bring it to a potluck. Please do everything you can not spread your germs to others.

SICK CHILDREN

This can be another "sore" spot. Children get sick a lot. Moms and dad must work. That means if your child is sick, as long as they can walk and are not running a high fever, they usually end up in school or daycare. Once again, honesty is the best policy. If possible, keep your sick child home. All parents who work should have a back up babysitter to care for sick children. Yes, it is an inconvenience and it can cost money. Think about it. Do you want your child exposed to sickness at school or daycare? Probably not. So please keep that in mind when sending a child out. Also, skip birthday parties and other social activities until your child is no longer contagious.

POOR DIET

As we mentioned above the immune system needs a clean diet. We suggest you avoid sugar. Ridding sugar from your diet is a major step to good health. You do not have to quit all at once. Keep a log for one week, writing down each time you eat processed sugar. You do not need to write down how many teaspoons or grams, just how many times you ate sugar. If you eat a candy bar, that counts as one. Ate a piece of cake? That counts as another one. At the end of the week count how many you had. Then decide to have less the next week. If you are a big sugar eater, you might want to drop 5-10 sugar eating instances. If your count for the week is 20 or less you might want to drop 1-3. Keep keeping track until you have quit.

Healthy eating

Following are just a few ideas toward healthy eating.

- Choose whole foods instead of processed.
- Do not drink sugary drinks, sodas, or caffeine drinks.
- Keep healthy food readily available.
- Eat whole grains and nuts
- Eat on smaller plates to reduce portion size
- Avoid red meat and pork
- Use organic ingredients if possible
- Avoid GMO
- Stay away from fast foods
- Plan your meals ahead of time
- Stay hydrated

There is plenty of information on the internet and at the library to help a person eat a healthy diet. Get rid of the chips, cookies and sodas in the house, so you are not tempted to eat them.

Take one step at a time. Do not overwhelm yourself (Yoder, 2017).

Chapter 4.

Finances

We have all heard that we should have three months of income saved in case of emergency. For those of us who live paycheck to paycheck, putting money aside for emergencies is nearly impossible. Do your best to stash away some extra cash. When you get paid, pay yourself before paying anything or anyone else, even if it is $5.00, it will add up in time.

Work

As we stated before work can become a challenge. Before a pandemic takes place, do what you can to find a part-time avenue to work at home in case of emergency. This is not possible for everyone, but if you can it will help, especially if you are not sick, but quarantined or must stay home to take care of a family member.

THE BILLS

The first thing you should do is call all your lenders and let them know the circumstances. Some will allow you to skip payments during times of disaster or sickness. If possible, try to get a month ahead on payments. It is more fun to buy something we would like to have or go out to a nice restaurant when we get a little extra money, but in the long run not having to worry about the bills for a month is can also be very rewarding.

Money for Supplies

If you have not already started putting extra supplies away, and do not have extra money for any, simply do your best. When you go to the store look for the two for one special and put one aside. Buy some sale items to put in the pantry. Do you have a health savings card that allows you to buy over the counter medical supplies? Use it. A little can add up to a lot over time.

CHAPTER 5.

SUPPLIES

One thing we all can do is make certain we have enough essential foods and goods on hand. As we stated in the previous chapter, you do not have to run out and buy it all at once. Just start today buy adding a little at a time. Look around your house and take stock. What do you have? What would you need if you must stay put for 14 days or more? Remember, stores shelves might be bare, gas pumps may not be working and delivery services may not be operating. Buy extra things you use now and rotate so nothing gets stale dated.

The following list is some of the things we need to stock up on:

- Extra prescription drugs
- Over the counter fever and pain medications

- Mucinex or other brand of mucus and congestion relief
- Feminine hygiene products
- Toilet Paper
- Paper Towels
- Tissues
- Soap
- Bleach
- Hand Sanitizer
- Household Cleaning Products
- Paper Plates
- Paper Cups
- Plastic Utensils
- Diapers and formula if you have a baby
- Games in case the grid goes out.
- Alternative cooking supplies, such as a grill and charcoal.
- Flea protection for pets
- Kitty Litter
- Contact lens solution

FOOD

- Cereals
- Grains
- Beans
- Lentils
- Pasta
- Tinned or packaged fish, chicken, veggies and fruit
- Oil
- Spices
- Dried Fruit and Nuts
- Powdered milk
- Food for pets
- Protein Bars
- Protein Powder
- Peanut or Almond Butter
- Soups
- Crackers

FOR THE CAR

It is important to keep the tank full. If we are quarantined it may be difficult to obtain fuel.

OTHER IMPORTANT ITEMS TO HAVE ON HAND

- Emergency cash
- Copies of important documents
- Flashlights
- Batteries
- Radio
- Plastic sheeting and duct tape
- Garbage bags with ties
- List of emergency contacts
- Matches, lighter

- Manual can opener

- Camping lights

- Candles

CHAPTER 6.

FIRST AID

Always keep a first aid kit available in your home and car. A conventional first aid kit is not enough if we are homebound and unable to go out for days. Following are recommendations to have on hand:

- Extra prescription medications
- Face masks, disposable gloves
- Hand sanitizer
- Alcohol
- Eye protection
- Hand sanitizer
- Cleansing wipes
- Water—at a minimum stock one gallon per person per day. In times of illness, you will need more!
- Drinks that contain electrolytes

- Over the counter, essential prescriptions and antivirals for a month (Discuss your options with your doctor)
- Blankets
- Copy of your health records
- Disposable gloves
- Masks. Masks are helpful, but standard surgical masks don't do much to fight the flu, because the virus is small enough to pass through. The CDC writes in its H1N1 flu advisory, "facemasks help stop droplets from being spread by the person wearing them. They also keep splashes or sprays from reaching the mouth and nose of the person wearing them. They are not designed to protect against breathing in the very small particle aerosols that may contain viruses."
- Household Bleach
- Cleansing wipes
- Soap

- Bandages, gauze and other wound care supplies
- Aspirin
- Ibuprofen
- Peroxide
- Saline Solution
- Ice packs

THERMOMETER

Whether it's caused by the flu or a common cold, having a fever is never fun. When your body temperature spikes, it's time to reach for a thermometer to understand just how bad the situation really is.

Thermometers have come a long way since the mercury-filled glass thermometers many of us used in the past. In todays world there are smart thermometers that can connect to an app to track your temperature over time, giving you a holistic view of your health. They're exceedingly accurate, and many of them offer an instant read. No matter how you want to take your or your child's temperature -- orally, on the forehead, in the armpit, in the ear -- there's a model out there for you.

For emergencies make certain you choose a thermometer that can be used without being hooked up to a computer or phone.

CHAPTER 7.

SANITATION

When a person is sick with the flu, there are a lot of germs to be found in body fluids. It is important to keep sanitation in mind.

The flu spreads when the sick person coughs, sneezes or even talks, affecting people as far as 6 feet away! Flu germs are also spread by touching a surface that has flu viruses on it. That's why we should keep the sick person confined to one room and one bathroom. It reduces exposure to the rest of the family and limits the number of rooms you must disinfect.

Disinfecting should be part of your usual cleaning routine, whether anyone at home is sick.

When using a disinfectant, check the label to make sure the disinfectant works against the viruses you're targeting, such as cold and flu viruses,

When you use disinfectant sprays, use paper towels. Disposable disinfectant wipes are best. Rags, dishcloths and sponges can spread germs. With paper towel you are spraying and then wipe the surface off. When using a disinfectant wipe the disinfectant stays on the surface until dry and that gives it more time to kill germs. It also leaves some residual impact.

Another option is to disinfect hard surfaces by wiping or mopping with a solution of 1/2 cup of bleach per gallon of water. Allow the solution to be in contact with the surface for at least five minutes. Rinse and air-dry.

Take care not to spread germs unintentionally. After mopping floors in the contaminated room and the designated bathroom, disinfect the mop head by soaking it for 15-20 minutes in a solution of 1/2 cup bleach and one gallon of water. Also, do not re-use cleaning cloths in other parts of the house. Toss them in the washer instead.

To sanitize kiddie items such as non-electric plastic/metal toys, sippy cups, teething rings, bottle nipples and dishes, wash items first then soak them for two minutes in a solution of 2 teaspoons of bleach per gallon of water. Rinse in warm water then air dry (Fields, n.d.).

WHAT TO DISINFECT

- Disinfect what people touch the most:
- Phones
- Computers – keyboards and screens
- The bathroom
- Faucets
- Light switches
- Land lines

- Towels (do not share towels or bed linens with those who are ill)
- All tables including play tables
- Toys and stuffed animals
- Bedding
- Floors
- Tabletops
- Countertops
- Remote control
- Doorknobs
- Sinks
- Tub
- Toilet
- Toilet handle

A sick person's towels, bedding and clothes (and the clothes of the caregiver, too) are full of germs, so don't "hug" dirty clothes as you take them to the washer. This could spread the germs onto you. Instead, transport dirty clothes in a laundry basket and wash your hands after loading the washer (Fields, n.d.).

CHAPTER 8.

WATER

To stay healthy, we need to drink plenty of water. We also need water for sanitation Storing water is very different from storing food. Water storage needs to be protected against viruses, bacteria and contamination. Different measures must be taken to protect your water from these threats than you would with food.

Water does not expire. It can become contaminated (chemically or biologically), but it doesn't "go bad." Water can have a stale taste, but that taste can be eliminated by rotating your water and purifying it. If a water storage source is in ideal conditions (if it started out clean and was stored in a dark, cool area, not directly on concrete or near harsh fumes and chemicals), it technically can store indefinitely.

Containers. Water should be stored in a UV-resistant, food-grade plastic container or in metallized bags. Traditionally, water storage barrels are blue. This color limits light exposure and biological growth (bacteria and algae) and signifies that what is stored in the container is safe for human consumption (for example, gasoline is stored in red containers).

Don't use milk jugs for water storage. Since milk jugs are biodegradable, they will break down over time. Also, any live cultures in the milk that remain in your jug could make you ill if you store drinking/cooking water in milk jugs.

You can't solely rely on the barrel for all the situations you may encounter. If you must evacuate, you won't be able to carry a water barrel with you. Also, if you only have one barrel or one water source you may run out of water given the number of people in your family and the number of days that you will be without water. Remember that the average amount of water to store is one gallon per day per person for a 2 week period.

Store water in various sized containers and plan for different situations (grab-and-go, shelter-in-place, extra water for cooking, etc.). You can siphon the water from your barrel into other containers and refill it before emergencies arise.

Water barrels are safest if they are stored standing. However, **do not store your barrel directly on cement or on the floor in your garage.** Plastics absorb flavors and odors from gasoline, liquids spilled on the floor, and chemicals used to create the concrete. These chemicals and odors will make the taste of the water unbearable to drink. Instead, place your water barrel on top of a wood board or cardboard so that odors and chemicals do not leach in.

Boiling

Often when a community water supply has been compromised, officials will issue a "boil order," advising everyone to boil water (a full, rolling boil) for at least one minute before using it to drink, cook, wash dishes, wash the face, or brush teeth. Boiling water from a natural source is effective, too, killing both bacteria and viruses. (This can take longer in high elevations where water boils at a lower temperature) (Essentials, 2013).

There are several companies that water filters can be bought from. We recommend "Life Straw" for on the go. They can be found on the internet. The official webpage is https://www.lifestraw.com/

WHAT TO DO WITH THE "DOO-DOO"

You'll want to add an emergency toilet to your disaster kit. In natural disasters the public sewage system can go down. In a pandemic, parts may not be available to keep things flowing.

One suggestion we found is to line a bucket with a heavy-duty 13-gallon garbage bag and then cover each use with sawdust, shredded paper, or grass clippings to help dry the excrement. Start a new bag when the poo bucket is half full. It is best to use a two bucket system. The buckets keep poo and pee separate. This minimizes volume and odor. It also makes it safer and easier to store and dispose of poo. Urine can be poured out into the yard.

For solid waste, a small amount of disinfectant can be added to the bag after use, if available. Diluted liquid chlorine bleach at a 1:10 bleach to water ratio, or powdered, chlorinated lime are suitable disinfectants. After use, remove the bag, seal or tie it closed, and carry it outside and place in a closed container away from people. Keeping a small bucket next to the toilet will make carrying the bag outside easier! Human waste should not be disposed of with regular the trash; however, a heavy duty trash bag can be used to line a trash can and all waste bags placed inside the larger bag, or one bin can be designated for human waste. If multiple bins are available label appropriately. Hopefully your city will later provide a means for disposing of this waste.

Digging a latrine or a pit toilet could be an option for people with big yards. It is suggested that the spot should be at least 10 feet from the property line and 100 feet from any stream or water source (Banse, 2018).

CHAPTER 9.

TRAVEL

Whether to travel when there is a pandemic scare is up to the individual. You'll want to read up before you travel on what, if any, policies all the countries you'll pass through have in place in terms of controlling the virus. You'll also want to know your own country's policy on people who have visited places with coronavirus outbreaks.

Are there any travel restrictions or advisories? If you go to a particular country and there's an outbreak or you catch the virus, can you get home? Does the country repatriate citizens? Would the country you're visiting quarantine you if you happened to have been in another country where the virus is spreading?

You will need to think about the uncertainties such as if you will able to handle a two week or more delay before getting home if you are quarantined. Also, you need to be certain you trust the countries you are traveling to will quarantine you safely. Will your insurance company cover you if you are hospitalized in the country you are traveling to?

The best advice about traveling is to gather as much information as possible. Do not rely on the news or gossip.

If you travel using hotel rooms wipe everything down, don't sleep with the comforter on bed (they rarely wash them) on the airplane wear mask, wipe down seats, and arm rests.

Chapter 10.

EMF

EMF is short for electromagnetic field. We are exposed to them every day. What happens when you are exposed to electromagnetic fields?

Exposure to electromagnetic fields is not a new phenomenon. However, exposure has been increasing steadily in the 20th century. Now with 5G we are being bombarded with these damaging frequencies. To keep our immune systems healthy, we must be aware of the dangers and do what we can to combat the damage they are causing.

Nearly everyone on the planet is exposed to a complex mix of weak electric and magnetic fields, both at home and at work, from the generation and transmission of electricity, domestic appliances and industrial equipment, to telecommunications and broadcasting (World Health Organization, 2019).

There is much to be told about how our bodies react to EMF. To keep things simple, we are going to give you some information and advise. Hopefully, you will educate yourself more in depth about the dangers.

Electric Fields

Low-frequency electric fields influence the human body just as they influence any other material made up of charged particles. When electric fields act on conductive materials, they influence the distribution of electric charges at their surface. They cause current to flow through the body to the ground.

Low-frequency magnetic fields induce circulating currents within the human body. The strength of these currents depends on the intensity of the outside magnetic field. If sufficiently large, these currents could cause stimulation of nerves and muscles or affect other biological processes (World Health Organization, 2019)

We personally watched the United States Congressional Hearings on 5G and what we heard was alarming. Doctor after doctor testified regarding negative health effects. In the end, those in favor of 5G had no studies providing any information.

CELLPHONE AND TABLET

To protect ourselves from the harmful effects of cellphones, we use EMF shields. These devices come in several sizes and you can stick them on your phone and tablets. Some work on quantum physics. Please be careful when choosing. One way to make certain they work is to purchase an EMF meter to measure before and after installation. It is good to measure the levels of radiation within 100 feet of your home. Research all the consumer products in this category so that you can protect yourself as much as possible.

Take some time away from your electronics. Abstain from using your cell phone for long periods of time, **including never keeping your cell phone in your bedroom**. If possible, keep your mobile devices five to ten feet away from you. When traveling with your cell phone, store it in an EMF protective bag.

Certain crystals are helpful. Orgonite, which reportedly scatters electromagnetic fields and turns them into beneficial ones. (Wagner, 2020). Orgonite is a composite developed by the late Dr. Wilhelm Reich. This composite can change harmful electromagnetic fields and transform them into harmless beneficial fields. It accomplishes this by emitting negative ions into the environment. You can place orgonite on your body, around your home, office and garden to protect you.

Elite Shungite is an equally powerful, EMF resistant stone. Shungite attenuates electromagnetic emissions from electrical grids, computers, cell-phones, Wi-Fi, appliances, and other electronic devices—meaning shungite transforms harmful manmade EMFs into wave forms that are more compatible with our biology." It can purify water. This is all due to the crystal's carbon content. Shungite is the only known natural mineral to contain fullerenes, a crystalline form of carbon. Fullerenes is an antioxidant that neutralizes free radicals. Fullerenes are anti-everything harmful to us including viruses, bacteria, fungus, pathogens, and all those harmful chemicals we are exposed to daily like fluoride and chlorine in our drinking water, to name a few. Shungite is an ancient stone, believed to be almost 2 billion years old. Shungite was formed when there were no life forms on earth, deep within the earths crust. The main deposit of Shungite on earth comes from the Zazhoginskoye deposit near Lake Onega in the Shunga region of Karelia, North West of Russia,

All computers, tablets, cell phones should have a blue light protector. To avoid macular degeneration. You can find these on Amazon or Ebay.

Be careful where you live. Avoid living near a cell tower or power station. (Wagner, 2020)

CHAPTER 11.

COMMUNICATION

Make a plan in case family members and close friends are quarantined. Keep in close communication. The biggest question to keep in mind is "What if?" and then plan for it.

Create a paper copy of the contact information for your family and other important people/offices, such as medical facilities, doctors, schools, or service providers. Make sure everyone carries a copy in his or her backpack, purse, or wallet. You should also post a copy in a central location in your home, such as your refrigerator or family bulletin board. If you are using a mobile phone, a text message may get through when a phone call will not. This is because a text message requires far less bandwidth than a phone call. Text messages may also save and then send automatically as soon as capacity becomes available.

Life disruptions can happen quickly during work or school hours. Discuss with your family members who could pick them up in an emergency. Make certain family members with phones are signed up with alerts and warning from their school, workplace and local government.

POLICE SCANNER

Scanners, commonly called "police scanners," are radio receivers designed to tune to radio frequencies used by police, fire, ambulance and a wide variety of other emergency services. There are phone apps that broadcast these frequencies. Listening to the police scanner during an emergency is a good way to keep informed.

CB RADIO AND WALKIE TALKIES

CB radios are capable of operating at a longer distance. If a walkie-talkie works at a distance of up to two miles, a CB radio is able to work at a distance of up to 20 miles. This is a significant difference in the range of the two devices. That doesn't mean a CB radio is better than a walkie-talkie. They are used in different situations. If your children are playing in the neighborhood, they do not need a CB radio. If you are on the road, a walkie-talkie would not be very useful. You would only be able to connect with neighboring cars and not with a more distant city. (SPRANDIN, THOMAS, 2020)

There is a minimum of two similarities:

- The transceivers are similar in appearance in both devices
- They both have channels.

Although both radios operate at different frequencies, they work within the spectrum of radio waves.

Walkie talkies work best for a small individual group. CB radios work between any with a CB within distance.

CHAPTER 12.

STAY CALM AND KEEP THIS BOOK HANDY

Fear only makes matters worse. Taking charge of any situation can eliminate it. Research has shown that different threats push different psychological buttons. Exotic threats pandemics raise anxiety levels higher than more familiar threats do. Experts agree that giving people concrete, detailed actions to take can help reduce panic and overreaction when a new threat emerges. Preparation is a key tool in decreasing situational anxiety such as fear of a pandemic.

Most importantly, keep practicing the coping skills you utilize all year long to manage your any fear you may have in regard to a pandemic or any life disruption. It's not out of the norm to have anxiety around the possibility of getting sick but try not to let that fear interrupt your day-to-day life. Taking small measures to reduce your anxiety about the flu can go a long way. Following are some ideas:

Meditation

Meditation is a wonderful practice that we urge all people to learn about and incorporate into their daily lives. Meditation is the practice of settling your mind through a conscious effort. The goal of meditation is for the mind to be quiet and free from stress through the use of contemplation and reflection.

Some physical benefits of meditation include:

- A decrease in blood pressure and an improvement in breathing.

- A lower resting heart rate and lower stress chemicals such as cortisol.
- Reduces stress: Stress reduction is one of the most common reasons people try meditation
- Controls anxiety
- Promotes emotional health
- Enhances self-Awareness
- Lengthens attention span
- May reduce age-related memory loss
- Can generate kindness
- May help fight addiction
- Taking small measures to reduce your anxiety about the flu can go a long way. There are many guided meditations that will help keep your mind focused.

EFT TECHNIQUE

Emotional Freedom Technique is a form of counseling intervention that draws on various theories of alternative medicine including acupuncture, neuro-linguistic programming, energy medicine and thought field therapy.

Yoga- a Hindu spiritual and ascetic discipline, a part of which, including breath control, simple meditation, and the adoption of specific bodily postures, is widely practiced for health and relaxation.

Tai chi- is an ancient Chinese tradition that, today ,is practiced as a graceful form of exercise, it involves a series of movements performed in a, slow focused manner and accompanied by deep breathing. Yoga includes various physical postures and breathing techniques, along with meditation.

Be proactive and reduce fear: Remain positive and strong, and continue to improve your health through positive thinking, forgiveness with increased attention toward mental, emotional, and physical health.

Love yourself and your family. Love has a profound effect on our health.

Earthing is a plus. Spend at least two hours in outside every week. Trees absorb our negative energies, improve our immune systems, and nourish our hearts and souls. Hugging a tree and walking barefoot in the woods can change your health, mind, attitude, thoughts, and intentions, and therefore, your current life-trajectory. Connecting with the earth in this way feeds our meridians and electromagnetic systems, which in turn can protect and empower us (News, 2019).

NET Therapy

NET stands for Neuro Emotional Technique. It is a safe, effective and natural way to instantly resolve long-standing health problems that have an emotional or stressful component. People used to think emotions resided entirely in their brain. Now we know other parts of the body can hold emotions too. Have you ever experienced butterflies in your stomach before a speech, referred to something as a "pain in the neck" or has felt a "lump in your throat". Clearly, emotions happen in our body, not just in our brain.

Most people say that would like to be healthy but something in their subconscious mind is not allowing this for them. So before you can become healthy that Neuro Emotional connection needs to be cleared. We find where the block is within the body and release it. The body is amazing and can heal itself when given the proper tools (Yoder, 2017).

Louise Hay wrote a book called Heal Your Body in which she states that mental thought patterns form our experiences. She believes that every illness or condition we have relates to a specific emotion and that once you heal that emotional issue, your body can heal itself.

We have noted some of the most common conditions and their related emotional issues that have come into our office.

These include:

• Ankles- inflexibility and guilt, ankles represent the ability to receive pleasure.

• Bunions- lack of joy in meeting experiences in life.

• Elbow- represents changing directions and accepting new experiences.

• Wrist- represents movement and ease.

• Hips- Fear of going forward in major decisions, nothing to move forward to.

• Knees- stubborn pride and ego, inability to bend, fear, inflexibility, won't give in.

• Neck- refusing to see other sides of the question, stubbornness, inflexibility.

• Shoulders- represent our ability to carry our experiences in our life joyously, we make life a burden by our attitude.

• Spine- represents the support of life.

• Lower Spine- fear of money, lack of financial support.

• Middle Spine- guilt, stuck in all that mess back there, "get off my back".

- Upper Spine- lack of emotional support, feeling unloved, holding back love.

- Arthritis- feeling unloved, criticism, resentment.

- Bone breaks/fractures- repelling against authority.

- Bursitis- repressed anger.

- Inflammation- fear, seeing red, inflamed thinking.

- Joints- represents changes in direction in life and the ease of these movements.

- Loss of Balance- scattered thinking, not centered.

- Sciatica- being hypocritical, fear of money and/or the future.

- Slipped Disc- feeling totally unsupported by life, indecisive

PRAYER

Prayer provides stress relief in a variety of ways. A prayer during these tense times relieves that feeling of loneliness. The belief that God is listening to our prayers and will help us is a source of hope to many individuals. With hope comes the strength to carry on.

Research shows that people who are more religious or spiritual use their spirituality to cope with life. Prayer can help us heal faster from illness and experience increased benefits of health and well-being. Spirituality enables us to stop trying to control things all by ourselves. It helps us feel part of a greater whole and understand that there is hope no matter what happens in life.

Make sure you have plenty of sleep every night. Relax and do not fear!

OTHER BOOKS BY THE AUTHORS- AVAILABLE ON AMAZON

Thinking Outside the Box – A Chiropractor's View to Alternative Healthcare – Dr. Patricia L. Yoder , 2017

Unimaginable Reality – Protect Your Child From Child Pornography, Child Trafficking and Exposure to Internet Pornography – Barbara Schneider MS, 2017

The Five Major Stressors to Your Body! Discovering the Sources of Hidden Toxins – Patricia L. Yoder, D.C. and Barbara J. Schneider MS

WORKS CITED

Banse, T. (2018, August 29). *Have You Planned For Number 2 After The Big One?* Retrieved from OBP: https://www.opb.org/news/articl e/emergency-toilet-disaster-preparedness-earthquake/

Banse, T. (2018, August 29). *Have You Planned For Number 2 After The Big One?* Retrieved from OPB: https://www.opb.org/news/articl e/emergency-toilet-disaster-preparedness-earthquake/

Branswell, H. (2020, February 12). *Understanding pandemics: What they mean, don't mean, and what comes next with the coronavirus.* Retrieved from STAT: https://www.statnews.com/2020 /02/12/understanding-pandemics-what-they-mean-coronavirus/

CDC. (2017, September 29). *Quarantine and Isolation.* Retrieved from CDC: https://www.cdc.gov/quarantine /quarantineisolation.html

CDC. (2020, February 14). *FAQS.*
Retrieved from CDC:
https://www.cdc.gov/coronaviru
s/2019-ncov/faq.html

CDC. (2020, February 24). *Legal
Authorities for Isolation and
Quarantine.* Retrieved from CDC:
https://www.cdc.gov/quarantine
/aboutlawsregulationsquarantine
isolation.html

Essentials, E. (2013, September 6).
*Making Water Drinkable: Ways to
Filter and Purify Water You Have
on Hand.* Retrieved from
https://www.beprepared.com/bl
og/9157/making-water-
drinkable-ways-to-filter-and-
purify-water-you-have-on-hand/

Fields, L. (n.d.). *Cleaning Hit List: What to
Disinfect.* Retrieved from Web MD:
https://www.webmd.com/cold-
and-flu/features/cleaning-hit-list

News, P. (2019, August 10). *How To
Protect Yourself From 5G And EMF
Radiation.* Retrieved from Planet
News:

https://www.planetxnews.org/ho
w-to-protect-yourself-from-5g-
and-emf-radiation/

Organization, W. H. (2019, November 7).
Electromagnetic fields (EMF).
Retrieved from World Health
Organization:
https://www.who.int/peh-
emf/about/WhatisEMF/en/index
1.html

Prevention, C. o. (2017, September 29).
Quarantine and Isolation.
Retrieved from CDC:
https://www.cdc.gov/quarantine
/index.html

Sprandin, Thomas. (2020, February 22).
Retrieved from Cozy Beat:
https://cozybeat.com/cb-radio-
vs-walkie-talkie/

Wagner, P. (2020, January 9). *How to
Protect Yourself from 5G and EMF
Radiation*. Retrieved from GAIA:
https://www.gaia.com/article/ho
w-to-protect-yourself-from-5g-
and-emf-radiation

Wikipedia. (2020, February 27). *Quarantined.* Retrieved from Wikepedia: https://en.wikipedia.org/wiki/Quarantine

Yoder, P. L. (2017). Totally Booked Practice. In P. Yoder, *Totally Booked Practice.*

NOTES

NOTES

NOTES

NOTES

NOTES